Loutfi Toumi
Mohammed Kara
Abdel jalil Senhaji

The effect of stimulant substances on the central nervous system

Loutfi Toumi
Mohammed Kara
Abdel jalil Senhaji

The effect of stimulant substances on the central nervous system

Cannabis and lysergic acid diethylamide (LSD)

ScienciaScripts

Imprint

Any brand names and product names mentioned in this book are subject to trademark, brand or patent protection and are trademarks or registered trademarks of their respective holders. The use of brand names, product names, common names, trade names, product descriptions etc. even without a particular marking in this work is in no way to be construed to mean that such names may be regarded as unrestricted in respect of trademark and brand protection legislation and could thus be used by anyone.

Cover image: www.ingimage.com

This book is a translation from the original published under ISBN 978-613-8-41854-2.

Publisher:
Sciencia Scripts
is a trademark of
Dodo Books Indian Ocean Ltd. and OmniScriptum S.R.L publishing group

120 High Road, East Finchley, London, N2 9ED, United Kingdom
Str. Armeneasca 28/1, office 1, Chisinau MD-2012, Republic of Moldova, Europe
Printed at: see last page
ISBN: 978-620-6-19958-8

TABLE OF CONTENTS:

CHAPTER 1   **3**

CHAPTER 2   **20**

CHAPTER 3   **29**

INTRODUCTION

According to the World Health Organisation, a drug is a natural or synthetic psychoactive substance administered by a person with the aim of altering their state of consciousness or improving their performance.

Psychoactive or psychotropic substances alter an individual's psyche and can affect perception, mood, consciousness, behaviour and various psychological and physical functions. They fall into five categories: central nervous system (CNS) depressants, CNS stimulants, CNS disruptors, psychotherapeutic drugs and androgens and anabolic steroids. Abuse of certain psychotropic drugs can lead to tolerance, psychological dependence, physical dependence and addiction.

Psychoactive substances exert their effects in the brain via different pathways. They associate with receptors that can increase or decrease neuronal activity, in this case that of the reward circuit.

The reward circuit is at the heart of our mental activity and guides all our behaviour. It's a complex circuit, but it has a central link that seems to play a fundamental role. This involves nerve connections between two small groups of specific neurons. One is located in the ventral tegmental area (or VTA) and the other in the nucleus accumbens. The chemical messenger that connects these neurons is dopamine. This is where most drugs act and produce dependence. (Ref. the brain at all levels).

In this dissertation, we focus on the study of two psychotropic substances that disrupt the functioning of the CNS and are classified as hallucinogenic, namely Cannabis, or Indian hemp, a plant grown in tropical or temperate regions and of which Morocco is considered to be one of the leading producers. From a legal point of view, it is classified as a narcotic but also has medicinal properties, and lysergic acid diethylamide (LSD), a powerful narcotic and hallucinogen.

How do cannabis and lysergic acid diethylamide (LSD) affect the CNS? What are their short- and long-term effects on human health?

CHAPTER 1

I. Cannabis :

1. History of cannabis :

Cannabis, or hemp, is one of the oldest plants known and cultivated by man, both for its agricultural value and for its medicinal and psychoactive properties. Some of its varieties are known as "Indian".

Its usefulness led to it being kept by all peoples through migrations from the central regions of Asia.

Today, it is found in almost every region of the globe, except in constantly cold regions or in primary rainforests.

The first evidence of the use of the Cannabis sativa plant, also known as Indian hemp, dates back more than 12,000 years (Abel EL. 1980).

In ancient times, it is highly likely that the inhabitants of Thebes were familiar with a cannabis-based sedative and analgesic potion as early as 4000 BC, and it is established that the Chinese have known about it for around 6,000 years, but it was not until around 1500 BC that the sacred books of Hinduism first mention the psychotropic properties of Indian hemp.

The history of therapeutic uses for cannabis is as old as humanity itself. But its modern history is highly unusual.

It can be traced back to the 1840s, when a young Irish doctor working in Calcutta rediscovered cannabis and began prescribing it to his patients suffering from rabies and rheumatism. (Mechoulam, R.; Hanus, L. A historical overview /2002)

From then on, the medical world became so passionate about this plant that from 1842 to the turn of the century, cannabis accounted for half of all medicinal sales, although by the end of the 19th century its medical use was beginning to decline.

It should be noted that this decline in popularity predates the wave of cannabis prohibition which began to spread throughout Western countries at the beginning of the present century (Journal de Pharmacie de Belgique 2002).

2. Description of the cannabis plant :

Cannabis Sative, the scientific name for Indian hemp, is an annual plant that can grow up to two metres tall.

It is a "Dioic" plant (from the Greek "Dis" meaning twice, and "Oikos" meaning house) (Hill R. J. 1983), which means a plant with two sexes: the stem of the plant can be male or female.

3

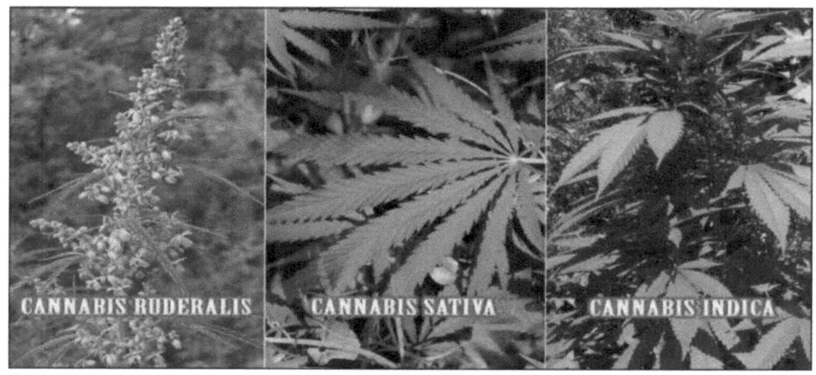

Figure 1: *Representation of the three cannabis species (https://notallowedto.com/new-specie-of-marijuana-discovered/)*

✓ **Botanical classification :**

Kingdom	*Plantae*
Subdomain	*Tracheobionta*
Division	*Magnoliophyta*
Class	*Magnoliopsida*
Subclass	*Hamamelidae*
Order	*Urticaria*
Family	*Cannabaceae*
Type	*Cannabis*
Species	*Cannabis sativa*

Figure 2: Cannabis classification (Vavilov, 1922) (http://www.wikiwand.com/fr/Chanvre_sauvage)

Both plants must be present for fertilisation. However, hermaphroditic plants can be found; the male plants are generally used for their fibres, while the female plants are cultivated to harvest their leaves, most of which contain psychotropic and medicinal substances (Hill R. J. (1983).

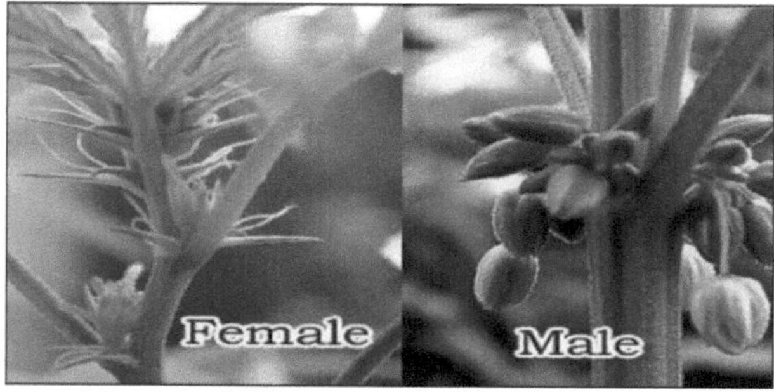

Figure 3: Representation of male and female cannabis plants.(http://fr.ilovegrowingmarijuana.com/comment-faire- grow-denorms-buds-marijuana/)

Cannabis leaves are characterised by 3 to 15 serrated fingers, each about ten centimetres long and one to two centimetres wide. Under the right climatic conditions, the plant can grow up to six metres tall.

All parts of the plant can be used. To do so, they have to undergo various processes. One of the first steps is to separate the chenvotte from the fibres, as these have different uses. (http://www.cannabis- medecin.fr/index.php/forms-consumed)
The various outlets for plant parts are shown in the diagram below.

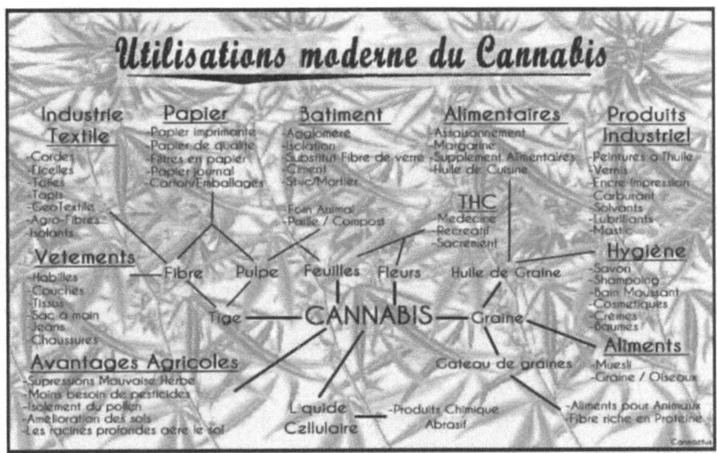

Figure 4: The different outlets for plant parts (http://geekmedia.over-blog.com/article-infographie-le-c-86888292.html)

3. Chemical composition of cannabis :

Numerous components have been described and isolated from hemp: essential oils; alkaloids; flavonoids; sugar; fatty acids; but the most important are the cannabinoids present in the leaves. These substances interfere with neurotransmitters and cause significant effects, although these vary according to their chemical properties (Meijer E. P. M. et al. 1992).

Approximately 75 types have been identified, divided according to their basic chemical structure into 10 main types: (ELSOHLY M. Marijuana and the Cannabinoids)

- Δ9-THC or Delta-9tetrahydrocanabinol
- CBC or cannabichromene
- CBD or cannabidiol
- CBL or cannabicyclol
- CBV or cannabivarol
- Δ9-THCV or tetrahydrocannabivarin
- CBDV or cannabidivarin
- CBCV or cannabichromevarine

5

- CBGV or cannabigerovarin
- CBG or cannabigerol

a. Cannabinoids: Tetrahydrocannabinol (A9-THC) :

In 1964, A9-THC was identified as the compound responsible for almost all the psychoactive properties of cannabis. It has the molecular formula $C_{21}H_{30}O_2$ and a boiling point of 157°C. It is a fragile thermolabile molecule that is easily isomerised into delta-8-THC (slightly less active) or transformed into cannabinol (particularly inactive) or cannabidiol (inactive).

A9-THC has a particularly low water-solubility, but is fat-soluble, which explains why it passes the blood-brain barrier so quickly and therefore has an almost immediate effect when consumed. This liposolubility means that it accumulates in fat, which explains why it remains present in the body for a very long time.

A9-THC binds mainly to cannabinoid receptors (CB1 and CB2) naturally present in the body, such as endogenous cannabinoid receptors (anandamide and arachidonic acid). These neurotransmitters belong to the endocannabinoid system, which is extremely important for the normal functioning of the body and is found in mammals and birds.

It plays an important neuroprotective role, and various in vivo and in vitro studies have shown that this system is capable of protecting neurons against various aggressions, such as excitotoxicity (excess glutamate release), as well as their role in regulating eating behaviour by reducing leptin (Dr. Nuss and others).

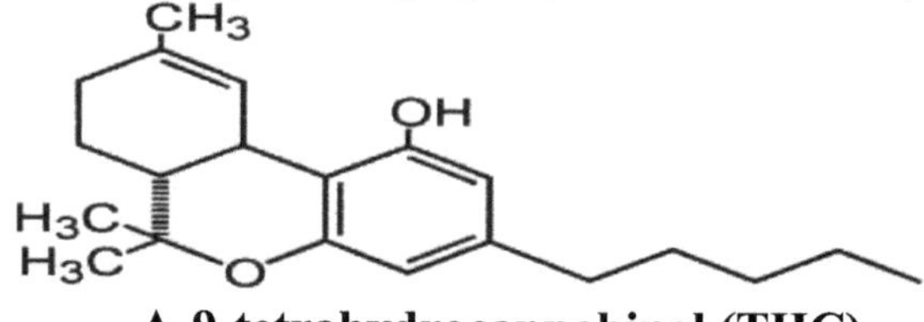

A-9-tetrahydrocannabinol (THC)

Figure 5: molecular structure of \9-THC

(https://cannabiscerveauetdependance.wordpress.com/2016/04/20/generalites-sur-le-cannabis/) Pr.Ferreri 2001)

b. Other cannabinoids :

- Cannabidiol :

Cannabidiol (CBD), the 2nd most studied cannabinoid after A9-THC, was isolated in 1940 by ADAMS and colleagues, but its structure and stereochemistry were determined in 1963 by Mechoulan. It has physicochemical properties similar to those of A9-THC.

CBD is hydrophobic and lipophilic, which means that it does not dissolve in water, but will dissolve in fat. It has significant medical benefits, according to several scientific and medical sources. Since 2013, the National Institutes of Health service

(PubMed) has included more than 1,100 studies on CBD in its database (Dr Nuss & Pr Ferreri 2001).

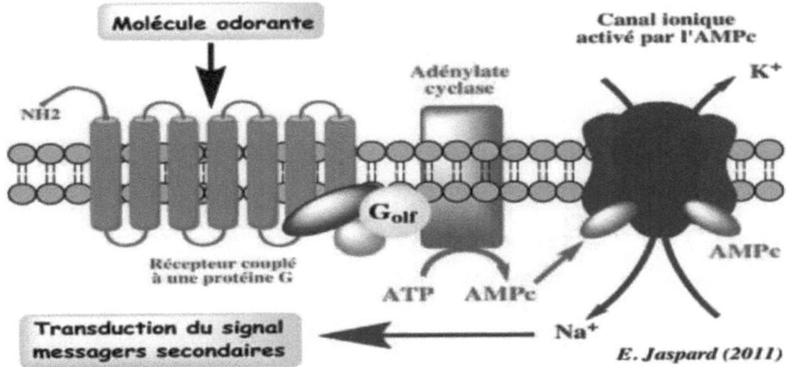

Figure 6: Molecular structure of CBD (Le Monde.fr 2014, "Le sativex médicament base de cannabis)

4. Mechanism of action of the active substance: A9-THC :
a. Cannabinoid receptors :

Cannabinoid receptors in the human body are known as CB1 and CB2. These receptors are differentiated by their action on the central (CB1) or peripheral (CB2) nervous system, and have in common the fact that they are stimulated as much by hashish and weed as by anandamide, (an endogenous cannabinoid par excellence) produced naturally by the body (Pertwee RG. 2001).

Figure 7: cannabinoid receptor coupled to G proteins (http://biochimej.univ-angers.fr/Page2/COURS/7RelStructFunction/2Biochemistry/5Signalisation/4RCPGetProteinsG/1RCPGetProtG.htm)

-Cannabinoid receptor (CB1) :

It is the most highly expressed cannabinoid receptor in the body and was discovered at the end of the 1980s by Devan and colleagues (WOOLRIDGE E., BARTON S.2005), who isolated the structure of the corresponding gene in 1990 and studied the distribution of A9-THC in the brains of rats. They observed that administration of A9-THC had virtually no effect on these mice: the compound had no receptor to bind to and consequently triggered no activity.

It is a protein complex composed of 472 amino acids, for a molecular weight of 67 KD that belong to the family of receptors 7 transmembrane helix is coupled negatively to a cyclase (SUGIUDE T., KISHIMOTO S., OKA S ET AL.2006) and positively to a protein kinase MAP KINASE. (PEREWEER.G, 2004)

This type of receptor is expressed by all organisms but is mainly found in brain regions involved in motor activities (cerebellar basal ganglia), memory (hippocampus, cerebral cortex) and pain signal processing (certain parts of the spinal cord) and in small quantities in a few peripheral organs that control energy balance at the metabolic level (adipose tissue; pancreas) as well as the salivary glands and certain parts of the organs of the reproductive system (SUGIUDE T., KISHIMOTO S.,OKA S ET AL 2006)

- **Cannabinoid2 (CB2) receptor :**

The discovery of the CB2 cannabinoid receptor followed that of CB1 and its structure was established by Munro et al in 1993. The CB2 receptor is also a protein complex of the 7 transmembrane helix family; linked to a GI protein and negatively coupled to adenyl cyclase, it is 44% common to the CB1 receptor (SUGIUDE T., KISHIMOTO S., OKA S ET AL 2006). The location of CB2 receptors is totally different from that of CB1; they are found in immune cells and lymphoid tissues such as the outer layer of the spleen, although they are rarely present at central level. (Dahchour A. Master P2Biomed Neuropharmacology, FSDM. Fès, 2016-2017)

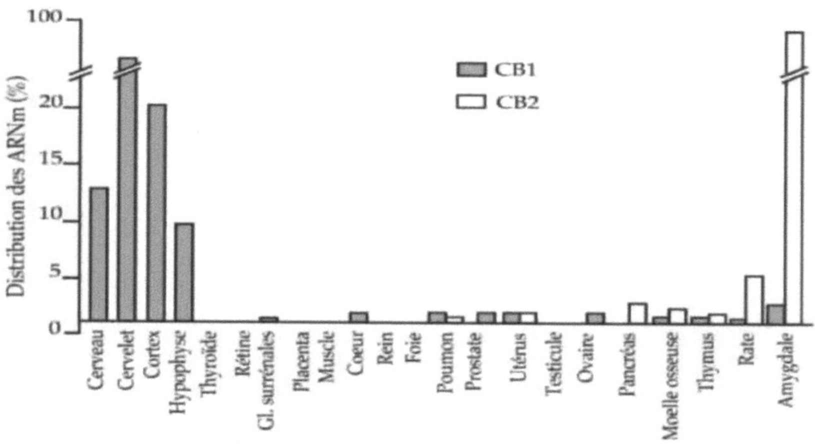

Figure 8: Distribution of CB1 and CB2 receptors in the body
(Ollat H, Pirot S. l. 2008)

Signal transduction mechanism :

We now know that the active ingredient in cannabis is Delta-9-tetrahydrocannabinol. Its presence intervenes in the reactions between neurons, known as synaptic reactions. In other words, A9-THC acts on the nervous system by interfering with synaptic reactions. In order to fully understand the changes caused by cannabis, we first need to explain how the nerves of an individual who does not use it work: But first, let's agree on a few words: b

A synapse is a functional contact zone between two neurons, or between a neuron and another cell (muscle cells, sensory receptors, etc.). It converts an action potential triggered in the presynaptic neuron into a signal in the postsynaptic cell. This is the most common type of neurotransmitter, using neurotransmitters to transmit information. (www.vulgaris- medical com/encyclopedie-medicale)

In the case of an individual who does not use cannabis: (Fig. 9)

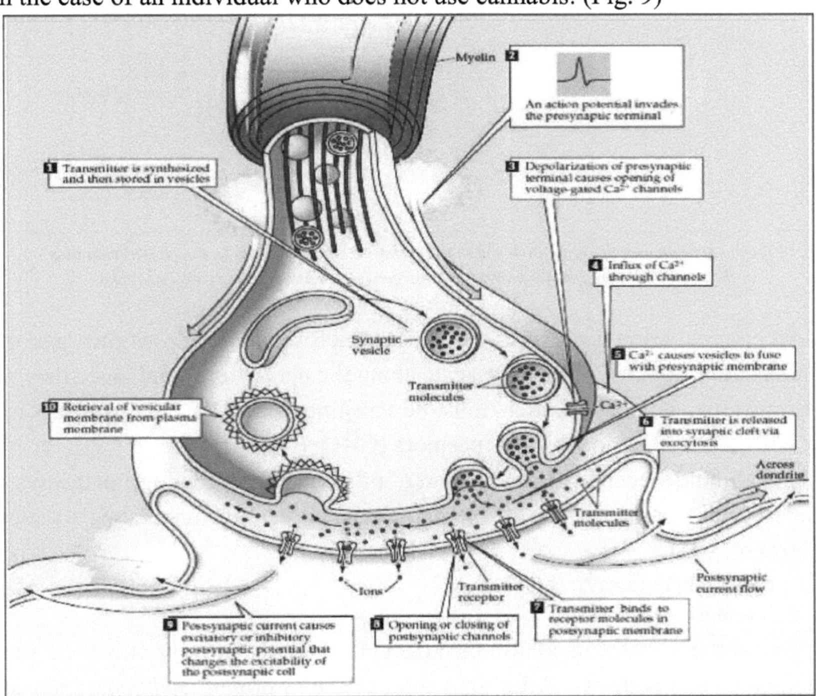

Figure 9: Sequence of events involved in nerve message transmission (Neuroscience Ed Dale Purves et al. 3rd Ed. 2004)

First of all, an external stimulus affects the organism, which sends a nervous message in the form of brief electrical signals, which travel along the nerve fibres and, once they reach the synaptic area, are transmitted to neurotransmitters. These neurotransmitters in the synaptic cleft. They bind to the post-synaptic receptors, which recognise the neurotransmitter that has bound and give the corresponding electrical signal frequency to the post-synaptic element. The nerve message is thus transmitted, the synapse has taken place. The neurotransmitters are then either destroyed by an enzyme designed for this purpose. Or recaptured by the presynaptic element via endocytosis vesicles specific to a single type of neurotransmitter. The synaptic cleft is clean and a new synapse can take place (www.vulgaris-medical.com/encyclopedie-medicale).

In the case of an individual who uses cannabis: (Fig. 10)

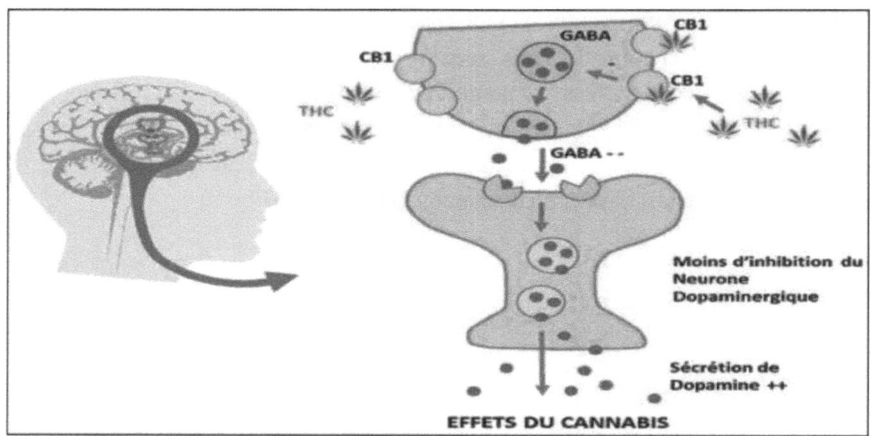

Figure 10: Sequence of events involved in nerve message transmission in the case of cannabis
(http://www.doctissimo.fr/sante/news/proteger-le-cerveau-des-effets-du-cannabis)

An external stimulus affects the body, which sends a nervous message in the form of electrical signals. These propagate along the nerve fibres and, once they reach the synaptic area, neurotransmitters must be transmitted. If A9-THC is present in this area, it will bind to the cannabinoid receptors (CB1). (Fig. 10)

cannabinoid receptors act on three intracellular signalling pathways: the adenylate cyclase pathway, the kinase pathway, and certain ion channels (calcium; potassium) for CB1.

- Signalling pathways: (Fig. 11)

➤ *Adenylate cyclase pathway :*

Cannabinoid receptors inhibit the adenylate cyclase pathway. It is the a subunit that modulates this pathway. After activation of the G protein and separation of the subunits, the a subunit inhibits adenylate cyclase, leading to a decrease in the level of cAMP (the second messenger) and inactivation of the PKA protein. This inactive PKA protein can no longer phosphorylate a number of components in the cell.

This lack of phosphorylation will have a number of cellular consequences, particularly in certain ion channels:

- the closure of calcium channels inhibits neuronal depolarisation.

- Opening potassium channels causes neuronal hyperpolarisation. This action on the ion channels has an inhibitory effect on the neuron, which no longer depolarises and therefore no longer releases neurotransmitters.

cannabinoids at the presynaptic level leads to a direct decrease in the levels of the most common neurotransmitters: glutamate, GABA (fig. 10), noradrenaline, dopamine, serotonin and acetylcholine. This intracellular signalling pathway is predominant for receptors located in the central nervous system (Venance Revue 2004).

➤ *MAP kinase pathway :*

The CB1 receptor activates the MAP kinase pathway. It would appear that this pathway is predominant outside the central nervous system. Although some of the consequences of activating this pathway are still unexplained, it has been shown that these receptors activate the intracellular MAP kinase cascade via a G protein, and that this effect is independent of the reduction in cAMP levels. The main consequence is the expression of several genes involved in the processes of cell survival, apoptosis, regulation of inflammation and cell proliferationIn   addition,   the   intracellular MAP kinase cascade activates

the Na+/H+ exchanger involved in protecting cells against acidosis and regulating pH and intracellular volume.

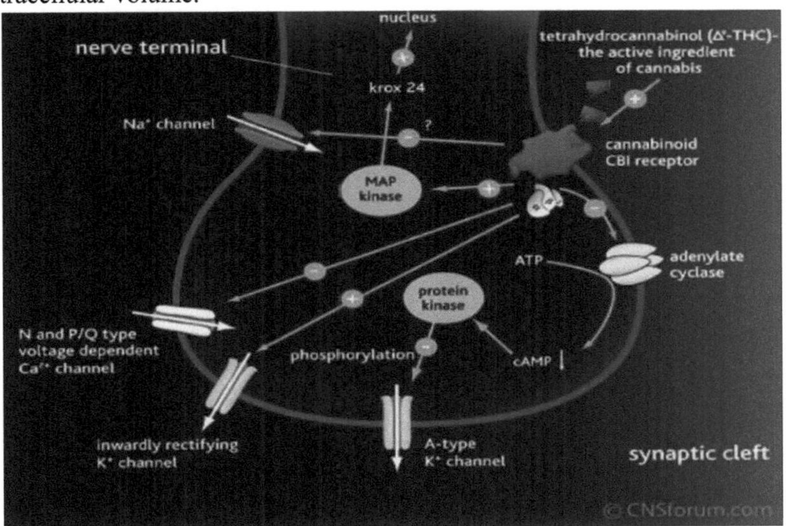

Figure 11: Action of &9-THC on synapse function
(http://healthmarijuanacanada.blogspot.com/2015_02_15_archive.html)

- **The action of cannabinoids on the reward system.**

The reward system is complex in humans, linking five different areas of the brain involved in pleasure sensations and social interactions (eating, feeding, defence, reproduction...).

These five zones interact with each other but all have specific functions, as listed below: (fig. 12)

The Amygdala: helps to assess whether an action is pleasurable or not, and whether or not it should be repeated.

The hippocampus: involved in recording memories associated with an experience/action.

The frontal regions of the cerebral cortex: coordinate and process all the information gathered previously and determine the individual's final behaviour.

The nucleus and the ventral tegmental area are linked by the mesolimbic circuit, which is responsible for informing its 3 partners (amygdala, hippocampus, cerebral cortex) and the hypothalamus of the importance of the reward.

We have focused on the action of cannabinoids on neurons in the ventral tegmental area and nucleus accumbens only. We will first explore the neurons of the ventral tegmental area and then those of the nucleus accumbens. (Venance Revue 2004)

The main effect of A9-THC is to intensely stimulate the reward system.

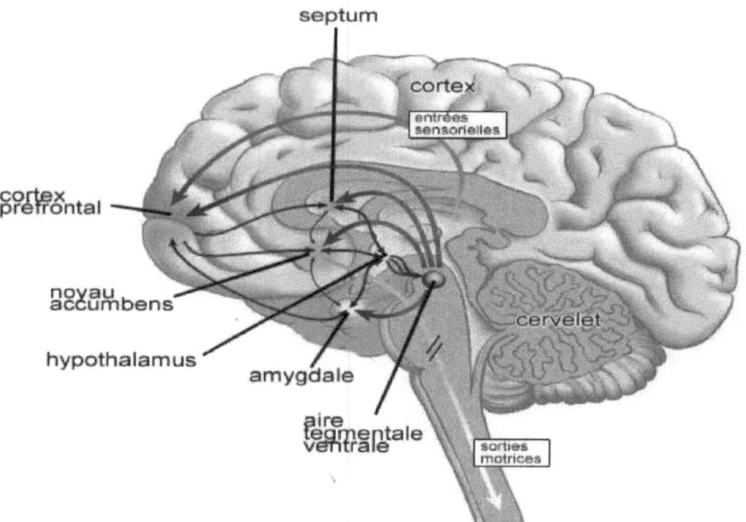

Figure 12: The reward circuit
(http://www.neuroperformance.fr/satisfaction-et-recompenses/)

Location of cannabinoid receptors: In the ventral tegmental area, there are GABAergic neurons that release GABA neurotransmitters, which have an inhibitory action, and in the nucleus accumbense there are dopaminergic (DA) neurons that release dopamine neurotransmitters.

(excitatory) neurons. GABAergic neurons are present upstream of the dopaminergic neurons. It is therefore the GABAergic neurons in the ventral tegmental area that regulate the release of dopamine from the dopaminergic neurons in the nucleus accumbense.

However, as with cannabis, there is an increase in the release of dopamine. Cannabis will therefore cause the inhibition of GABA neurons to be lifted by the binding of A9-THC to CB1, which is located on GABAergic neurons that induce their cascade of reactions and consequently activate dopaminergic neurons that have released dopamine, which will bind to its receptors located on the neuron of the nucleus accumbens and transmit its signal to this neuron, resulting in the individual experiencing a sensation of well-being (pleasure). (http://lecannabisdonnefaim. blogspot.com/p/laction-des-canabinoides-sur-le- systeme.html)

5. The effects of cannabis :

a. The short-term effects of cannabis :

The initial effects of cannabis depend on a number of factors. There are major differences depending on the individual, the product used (form and quantity) and the context of use. (Galland J-P, 1992)

Acute cannabis intoxication is mainly due to the effects of A9-tetrahydrocannabinol (A9-THC), although other constituents of the Cannabis sativa plant may also be responsible. The clinical symptoms presented by chronic users and due to the effects of the active substances in cannabis vary according to the way in which they are taken. (Etiemble J.2001)

The effects appear very quickly if cannabis is used by inhalation (a few minutes), with a maximum effect in 30 minutes and a duration of action of 2 to 4 hours. When ingested, the onset of action is slower, with the effects taking one to two hours to be felt. A study carried out on 880 students (average age: 20) and published in L'Encéphale (psychiatric medical community) in 2009, looked at the effects felt following the first doses of cannabis: (fig. 13) (Julienne M. 2013)

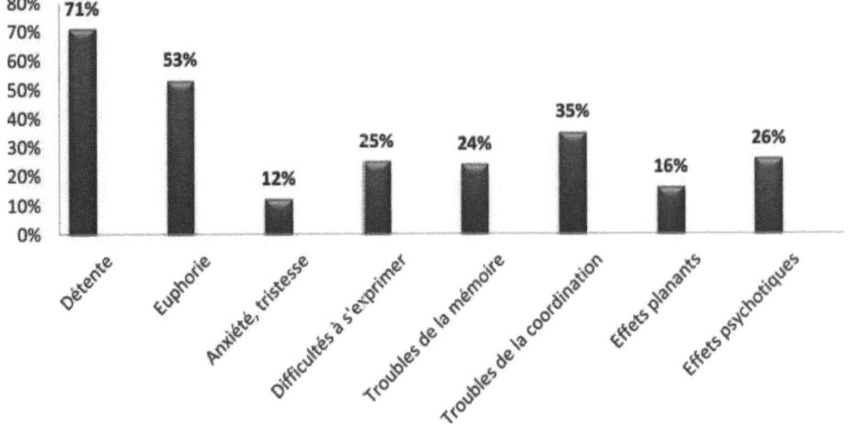

Figure 13: Effects felt when first taking cannabis (Julienne M. 2013)

- **Central effects of cannabis :**

These effects vary from one person to another. These effects vary from person to person, with some people experiencing euphoria very quickly and others falling into a state of sedation or even lethargy. Thymic disorders such as anxiety may also occur.

- **Peripheral effects :**

Prolonged use of cannabis can lead to symptoms of tachycardia, bronchodilation, red eyes and dry mouth.

The acute toxicity of cannabis is very low. The estimated lethal dose is 20,000 to 40,000 times the level of a normal dose, which would be equivalent to administering 681 kilograms of cannabis in 15 minutes. This is why cannabis is often referred to as a "soft drug", unlike "hard" drugs such as heroin or cocaine, where the risk of overdosing is deadly (Galland J-P. 1992).

b. The long-term effects of cannabis :

Long-term, chronic cannabis use can cause a host of health problems, and some of its effects are far from harmless or even harmful. Consumers expose themselves to numerous health risks, including circulatory and respiratory pathologies and certain mental illnesses.

- **Somatic complications :**

Cardiovascular complications are more closely linked to A9-THC. Studies show that it has a vasoconstrictor effect. It also reduces cardiac output and has an arrhythmogenic effect. Orthostatic hypotension has also been observed, and there is a possible link with arteritis in young subjects (cannabis is thought to be at least a contributing factor).

Oro-digestive complications Regular use of cannabis can lead to nicotine stomatitis. Daily use of cannabis can also cause cannabinoid hyperemesis syndrome: episodes of vomiting, nausea and abdominal pain.

The main mucocutaneous complication is frequent and repeated conjunctivitis. Cannabis also appears to be involved in allergic reactions such as asthma and urticaria.

There are also numerous gynaecological and obstetric complications. In women, chronic cannabis use leads to disruption of menstrual cycles, abnormal ovogenesis and the risk of retarded foetal growth.

In men, there is a reduction in sperm count and motility, with sexual problems such as erectile dysfunction and ejaculation. (Coscas S. Dec 2013)

- **psychiatric complications:**
- *Influence on motivation :*

In regular users, a drop in motivation or "amotivational syndrome" is observed, defined as an existential disinvestment. People with this syndrome experience an overall reduction in activities, psychological and physical asthenia, indifference and a lack of interest in professional activities. In addition, the person becomes withdrawn, with a risk of marginalisation and dropping out of school. Family and social life is greatly reduced

- *Cannabis and schizophrenia :*

Schizophrenia is a multifactorial illness. In predisposed individuals, cannabis is likely to reveal or aggravate manifestations of this serious mental illness. It is estimated that 8 to 10% of the population is "vulnerable", i.e. around 6 million people with a theoretical risk of becoming schizophrenic. Cannabis cannot therefore be held solely responsible. The risk of schizophrenia appears to be greater if cannabis use began in adolescence, and when such use is widespread. In addition, the relative risk of developing schizophrenia among cannabis users is multiplied by four (Julienne M.

2013) (Richard D, Senon J-L. 2010).

c. Cannabis tolerance and dependence:

Tolerance is defined as the need to increase the dose of a drug to obtain an effect that is quantitatively as strong as with a defined initial dose. In other words, you have to increase the dose more and more in order to achieve the same effect. Two hypotheses explain this mechanism:

- The body develops detoxification mechanisms that enable it to eliminate the substance more quickly, leading to more frequent consumption.

- Receptors to the drug become less sensitive, forcing the user to increase doses to stimulate them sufficiently.

As far as cannabis use is concerned, the development of tolerance has long been debated. Today it is accepted that tolerance does exist, but that it is low. Dependence on a drug is defined by the appearance of a withdrawal syndrome (= craving) when the drug is stopped, the appearance of tolerance, and the impossibility of abstaining from use. A distinction must be made between :

- ✓ physical dependence, resulting in the appearance of somatic problems (e.g. muscle cramps, tremors, hot flushes, sweating, gastrointestinal problems, etc.).
- ✓ psychological dependence, resulting in anxiety, anguish and irritability.

Because the tolerance and dependence associated with cannabis are low, it is considered a "soft drug", unlike heroin, which is highly addictive. (Richard D, Senon J-L. 2010) (Coscas S. déc 2013)

d. Cannabis antagonists :

- Action of pregnenolone to reduce the effect of cannabis :

In January 2014, two teams of INSERM researchers discovered that a molecule produced naturally by our brain, pregnenolone, protects us from cannabis intoxication (Protection naturelle contre le cannabis, 2014).

Pregnenolone was previously known as a precursor of steroid hormones (progesterone, testosterone, etc.). A new role has just been discovered for it by the Inserm teams: "pregnenolone constitutes a natural defence mechanism against cannabis and may protect the brain from the harmful effects of this drug".

The researchers demonstrated that over-activation of CB1 receptors by high doses of THC (higher than those to which regular smokers are exposed) triggers the synthesis of pregnenolone. Pregnenolone then binds to a specific site on CB1 receptors and reduces some of the effects of THC. This natural process protects the brain from over-activation of CB1 receptors.

In neurobiological terms, pregnenolone reduces the release of dopamine triggered by THC, and the excessive release of dopamine is considered to be the basis of the addiction phenomenon (for all drugs).

Identifying these mechanisms will enable researchers to develop approaches for treating cannabis addiction. However, the researchers are clear about the therapeutic use of pregnenolone: "This hormone cannot be used as a medicine as it is poorly absorbed and rapidly metabolised by the body". But "we have developed pregnenolone derivatives that are stable and well absorbed, and which in principle can be used as a medicine. We hope to start clinical trials soon to see if our expectations are confirmed and if we have truly discovered the first pharmacological therapy for cannabis dependence". (Piazza P-V 2014)

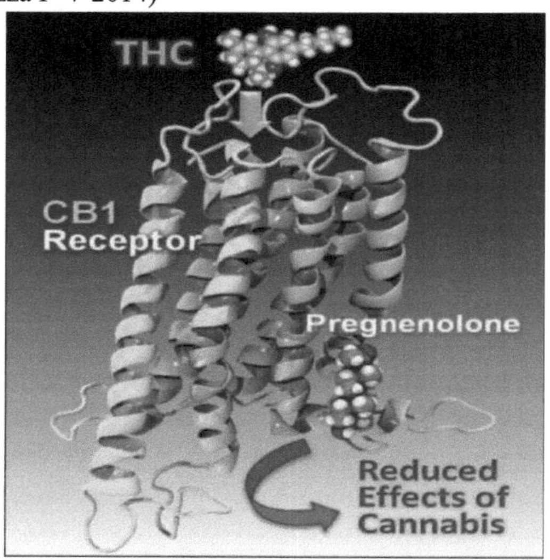

Figure14: Binding of pregnenolone to the CB1 receptor (P. Vincenzo Piazza and G. Marsciano, 3 January 2014).

6. The medicinal properties of cannabis derivatives:
a. Cannabinoids and the treatment of analgesic pain:

Pain is defined as "an unpleasant sensory or emotional experience associated with actual or potential tissue damage or presented in terms that describe such damage". There are two types of pain:

- Nociceptive pain (due to excess nociception): results from activation of peripheral pain receptors by an external pain stimulus.
- Neuropathic or neurogenic pain: this is linked to the destruction or lesion of a peripheral or central nerve structure, so the painful stimulus is internal. Cannabis is of interest in the treatment of chronic pain, particularly neuropathic pain. (Grotenhermen F. 2009) (2008.Clerc D)

What is the link between cannabis and neuropathic pain?

One way of reducing pain is to act on the release of endorphins. There is a feedback pathway made up of neurons from another region of the brain, the periaqueductal grey matter (PAG), which projects onto the spinal cord. These cells release endorphins at the axonal endings, which reduce pain (**Fig.15**).

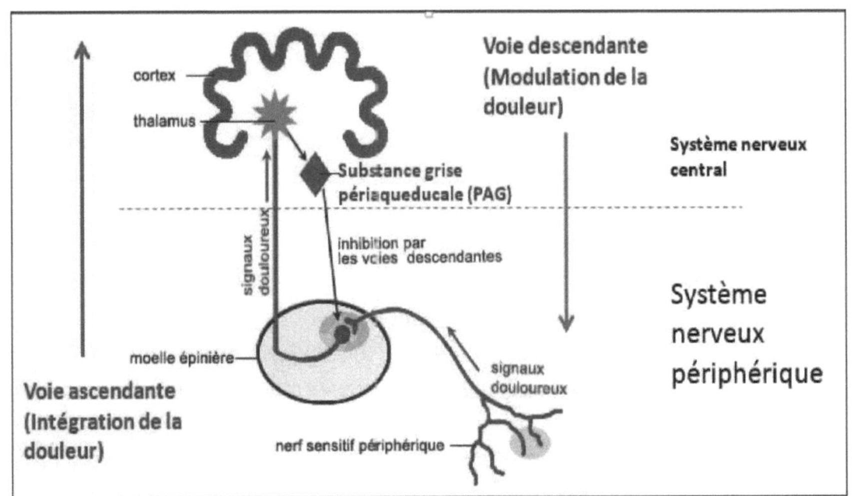

Figure15: feedback pathway between the brain and the spinal cord
(http://carayonbenjamin.wixsite.com/cannabismedecine/quest-ce-que-la-douleur-neuro)

Cannabis increases the release of endorphins and therefore has a significant analgesic effect (reducing the perception of pain).

This is because the PAG contains GABAergic cells which release GABA neurotransmitters. These cells inhibit the PAG cells that release endorphins. These inhibit the release of endorphins. GABAergic cells reduce pain inhibition.

CB1 receptors are present in the PAG, and more specifically on these GABAergic cells. When cannabinoids bind to these receptors, they inhibit these inhibitory cells. In this way, as if the brake had been removed, the PAG cells projecting into the periphery of the spinal cord will release large quantities of endorphins and relieve the pain. It therefore seems possible that CB1 can help the body to reduce this pain.

One of the mechanisms proposed by the scientists is that the activation of CB1 receptors increases the feedback pathway for pain inhibition induced by the endorphins released by the cells of the PAG at the level of its projections into the spinal cord. Cannabinoids therefore act in the brain, within the PAG, to increase the activity of these neurons and potentially increase the endorphins released.

GABAergic cells are inhibitory cells in the central nervous system. In AGP, these neurons inhibit the main cells by releasing GABA neurotransmitters. We know that CB1 receptors are present on the membrane of GABAergic cells.

The activation of CB1 by cannabinoids stops the release of GABA. As a result, the disinhibition of PAG cells potentially allows more endorphins to be released, which in turn inhibits pain, so that it is felt less. This is how cannabinoids play a role in the analgesia of neuropathic pain. (Ref : http://carayonbenjamin. wixsite.com/cannabismedecine/action-des-cannaïbinoides)

b. Cannabinoids and neurodegenerative diseases :

Alzheimer's disease :

Alzheimer's disease is a neurodegenerative disorder characterised by a progressive deterioration in memory and behaviour. The disease has a major impact on patients' quality of life: the progressive deterioration of intellectual functions leads to psychological symptoms and behavioural disorders, resulting in a loss of independence. The final stage is senile dementia.

Alzheimer's disease is the result of a pathological process which leads to the development of two types of lesions in the central nervous system:

- neurofibrillary degeneration: this is the appearance, within neurons, of abnormalities in the Tau protein, encouraging the production of hyper-phosphorylated Tau protein.
- amyloid plaques or "senile plaques": these are deposits of amyloid P protein outside neurons, produced by the cleavage of amyloid P precursor protein (APP) by P- and Y-secretases (Grotenhermen F. 2009).

Cannabinoids represent an interesting new therapeutic avenue for preventing or delaying the symptoms of Alzheimer's disease, as they act in different ways against this pathology: (Fig. 15)

By reducing the aggregation of beta-amyloid peptide plaques, the main marker of Alzheimer's disease, and by reducing the phosphorylation of
T au proteins, another biological marker of this condition.

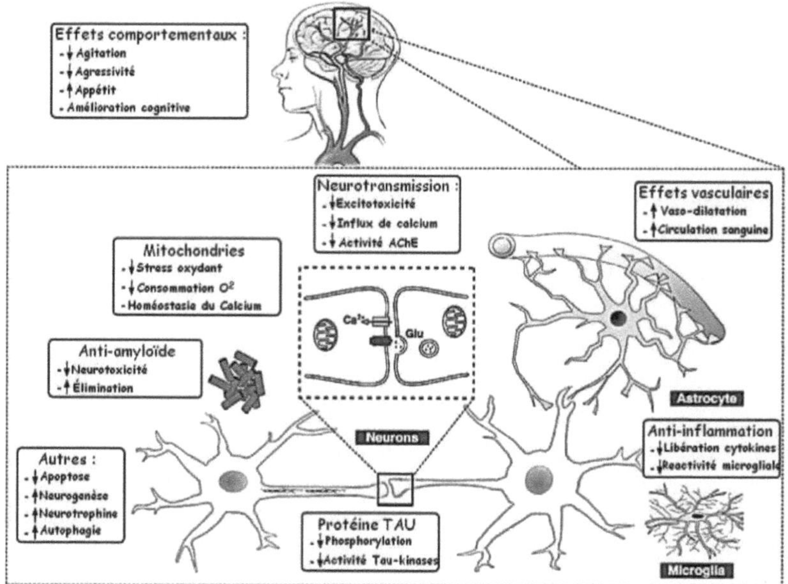

Figure 16: Effects of cannabis on Alzheimer's disease (https://www.alchimiaweb.com/blogfr/cannabis- contre-alzheimer/)

A 2005 study concluded that the administration of a non-psychotropic cannabinoid, cannabidiol (CBD), also reduced memory loss in a mouse model of the disease (Ramirez et al. 2005).

In 2006, a Californian study (Eubanks et al. 2006) showed that A9-THC inhibits P- and Y-secretases, the enzyme responsible for aggregating amyloid plaques. "Our results explain the mechanism by which the A9-THC molecule can directly influence the pathology of Alzheimer's disease", conclude the researchers. "A9-THC and its analogues may provide an improved therapeutic option for Alzheimer's disease by simultaneously treating the symptoms and progression of the disease".

Another study conducted in 2007 concluded that "cannabinoids offer a multifaceted approach to the treatment of Alzheimer's disease by producing neuroprotection and reducing neuroinflammation". (Campbell VA, Gowran A. 2007)

II. Lysergic Acid Diethylamide LSD :

1. Definition:

Lysergic acid diethylamide (LSD) is a substance obtained from a parasitic fungus, ergot. It is a very powerful hallucinogenic psychotropic substance that affects the central nervous system. LSD usually comes in the form of pieces of paper containing the substance, sometimes in liquid form or in tablet form. LSD use can lead to serious and irreversible psychiatric disorders. (Pierrick H, 2014)

The majority of hallucinogens are of plant origin, but the most powerful is a synthetic compound: lysergic acid diethylamide-25 (LSD), one of the most common drug psychedelic agents. The latter has been produced changes in perception, visual hallucinations, thought disorders and distortion of time, changes in the state of consciousness, euphoria, a feeling of positive mood; feelings of joy (Savage, C. 1952).

It stimulates the sympathetic nervous system, causing hyperthermia, sweating, palpitation, increased blood pressure, convulsions, increased muscle tension, tremors and muscular incoordination. (Goodman, N. 2002) (Schmid, Y.; Enzler, F,...2015)

2. History of LSD :

In 1918, the Swiss pharmaceutical company Sandoz isolated ergotamine, a compound found in ergot. In the early 1930s, American scientists defined the fundamental constituent structure of ergot: lysergic acid. In 1938, Albert Hofmann, a chemist at Sandoz, in turn synthesised a series of lysergic acid derivatives with the aim of developing drugs to regulate blood pressure or promote venous irrigation (CLERVOY Patrick).

A few years later, in 1943, during a re-evaluation of the product, Hofmann experimented with its effects after accidentally absorbing a low dose of LSD. He decided to test what he considered to be a low dose (250 micrograms) of LSD on himself (NORTIER E. 2007).

He left a description of his subjective experience and first voluntary 'trip' in the literature: "Phantasmagorical and colourful forms swept over me, transforming themselves like a kaleidoscope, opening and closing in circles and spirals, gushing out in fountains of colour, reorganising and intersecting, all in a constant stream. I noticed in particular the way in which all acoustic perceptions, such as the sound of a doorknob or a car passing in front of the house, were transformed into optical sensations. Each sound produced an animated image of corresponding shape and colour. (CHAPARD P. 2008)

He accidentally discovered psychological effects. Although he had synthesised numerous lysergic acid derivatives, none had the psychological effects aspect.

During the 1950s, LSD was presented to the medical community as an experimental tool for psychotic patients in the normal ("psychosis model") and later to improve psychotherapeutic treatments. (Passie T. 1997) (Abramson HA, 1967).

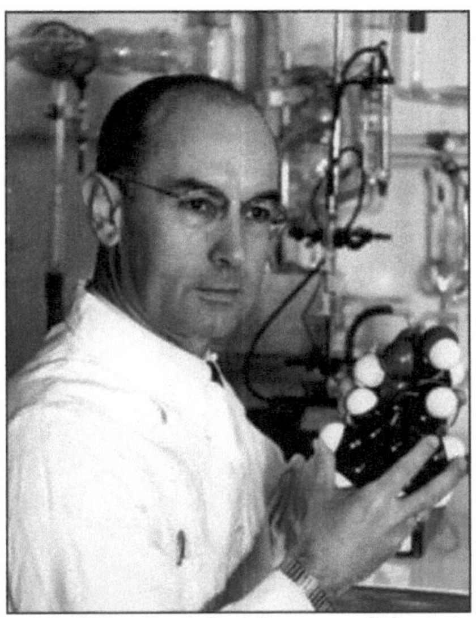

Figure 17: Hoffmann, 1938 and the LSD molecule (http://www.serendipite-strategique.com/exemples/lsd.html)

3. LSD derivative :

❖ **Rye ergot:** (*Claviceps purpurea*)

✓ **Botanical classification :**

Kingdom	*__Fungi__*
Branch	*Ascomycota*
Sub-branching.	*Pezizomycotina*
Class	*Sordariomycetes*
Subclass	*Hypocreomycetidae*
Order	*Hypocreales*
Family	*Clavicipitaceae*
Type	*Claviceps*

Non-binominal: Claviceps purpurea
Figure 18: Classification of rye ergot (Tulasne, L.R. (1853)

LSD 25 is an alkaloid from rye ergot. This fungus, Claviceps purpurea, is a parasite of cereals (particularly wheat and rye), responsible for ergotism epidemics. The cause of ergotism epidemics was recognised in the 12th century. The predominance of vascular or nervous symptoms now appears to be linked to the type of alkaloid contained in ergot.

These include water-soluble alkaloids of the LSD family, responsible for neurotropic symptoms (hallucinatory and delirious psychic disturbances, epileptic-type convulsions), and peptide alkaloids, responsible for vasoconstriction. The composition of ergot can vary considerably and the proportions of these two types of alkaloid differ to a large extent. (JUNGMANN C. 1997)

It consists of a mycelium (vegetative part of fungi). When the grains ripen, the filaments agglomerate into a dense tissue covered with a purplish bark visible to the naked eye, the sclerotia, which attaches itself to the grains of the cereal. Its pharmacologically active substances are ergoline alkaloids (Moyse H. 1976).

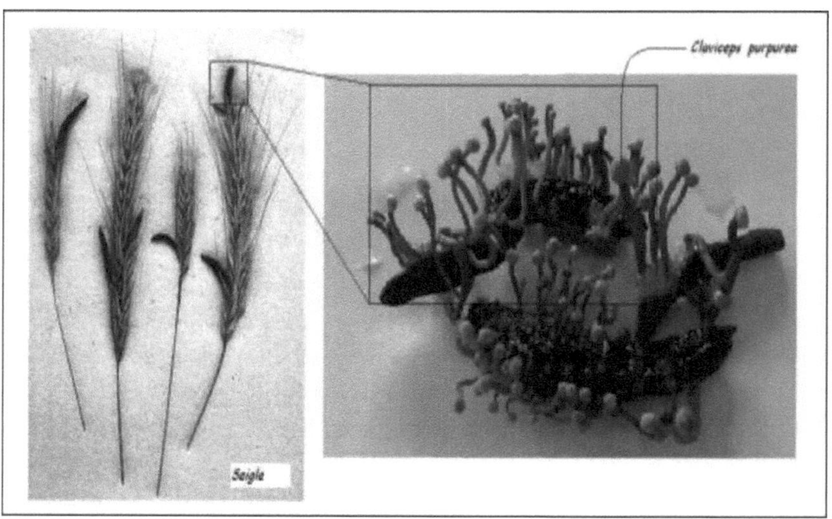

Figure 19: ergot fungus (http://tpelsd.e-monsite.com/pages/l-histoire-du-lsd.html)

Here we'll be looking at a synthetic derivative made by Albert Hofmann from lysergic acid: LSD 25 or lysergic acid diethylamide.

4. Epidemiology of LSD:

The overall prevalence of LSD use in Europe is generally low and has been stable for several years. For young adults (aged 15-34), the lifetime prevalence of LSD use varies from country to country.

In France, for example, LSD use among 17-year-olds in mainland France was stable between 2008 and 2011. (BASTIANIC T., BRISACIER A-C., CADET-TAÏROU A. et al/2013)

Between 2005 and 2010, experimentation with LSD among 15-30 year olds in France rose from 1.6% to 2.2% of the population, with three times as many men (3.2%) as women (1.1%) affected in 2010. Over the same period, LSD use has not changed, affecting 0.4% of 15-30 year-olds, with twice as many men as women.

In 2010, 2.2% of the French population aged 15-30 had experimented with LSD. Experimentation with LSD peaks among men aged 26 to 30, then declines in the 31-

64 age group. Between the ages of 15 and 64, young people aged 15 to 19 experiment the least with this synthetic drug. Current use of LSD is highest among men aged 20-25 and virtually nil among those aged 31-64 (BECK F., RICHARD J-B/2013).

In 2011, 1.3% of 17-year-olds had experimented with this drug, and the same trend as for 18-64 year-olds was observed: the frequency of experimentation declared by 17-year-old girls (0.9%) is still lower than that of boys (1.7%), but with smaller differences than among adults, probably indicating a generational change.

LSD is characterised by a significant increase in the level of experimentation, although this does not translate into an increase in use: Although their use is the hallmark of a passage through the party scene, hallucinogens also form part of the range of consumption of some of the often marginalised people who frequent reception and harm reduction facilities for drug users.(BASTIANIC T., BRISACIER A-C., CADET-TAÏROU A. et al/2013)

5. Structure and chemical properties of LSD :

❖ Lysergic acid diethylamide :

When Albert Hofmann first discovered lysergic acid diethylamide, he wrote down LysergSaureDiethylamid-25: LSD-25. Its chemical name is N, N-diethyl Dlysergamide, and its molecular formula is C20H25N3O.

LSD is an alkaloid derivative, which can be obtained from ergoline. It therefore has an indole-type aromatic heterocyclic ring, like many other hallucinogens (tryptamines, psilocybin, harmaline, etc.).

It is soluble in water and has a melting point of 83°C, as well as a molecular weight of 323.4 g/mol. It is very sensitive to air and light; in contact with oxygen in the air, it is decomposed by oxidation and in the presence of light, it is transformed into an inactive product. (Marie-Hélène GHYSEL, Francis TROTIN/2004)

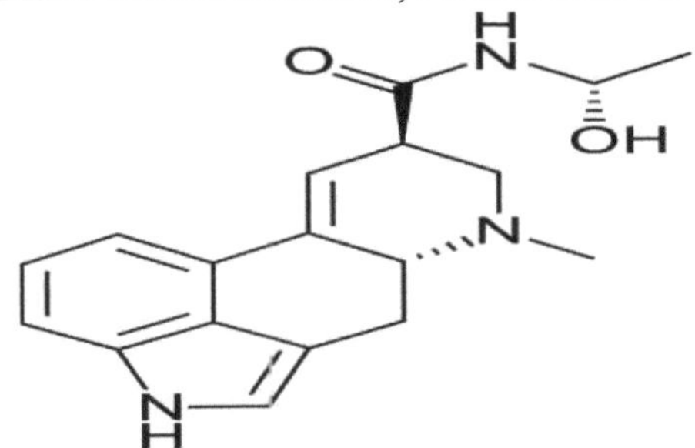

Figure 20: Molecular structure of lysergic acid diethylamide

(https://commons.wikimedia.org/wiki/File:Dlysergic_acid_methyl_carbinolamide.svg)

Mode of action of the active ingredient Lysergic acid Diethylamide

LSD has a molecular structure similar to serotonin, and acts specifically on 5-HT1 and 5-HT2 receptors (Marie-Hélène GHYSEL, Francis TROTIN/2004).

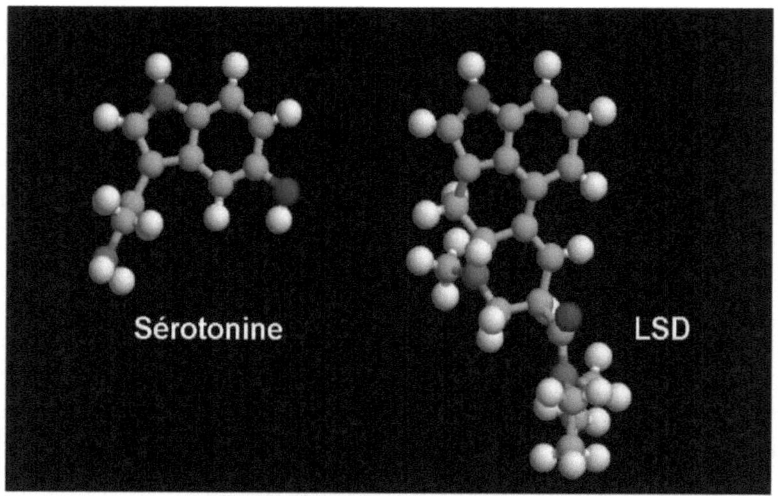

Figure 21: diagrams showing the serotonin molecule is LSD
(http:/raymond.rodriguez1.free.fr/documents/organisme-A/vision/lsd-serotonin.jpg)

a. 5Hydroxy-tryptamine1 and 5Hydroxy-tryptamine2 receptors:

- **5-hydroxy-tryptamine1A receptors (coupled to Gai) :**

5-HT1A receptors, composed of 422 amino acids, This class of receptors inhibits the activation of CA and the production of cAMP via the inhibitory protein Gai/o. Through the 0Y subunits of this protein, these receptors are responsible for opening K+ channels and reducing neuronal excitability, as well as closing Ca2+ channels and reducing neurotransmitter release (Nichols & Nichols, 2008).

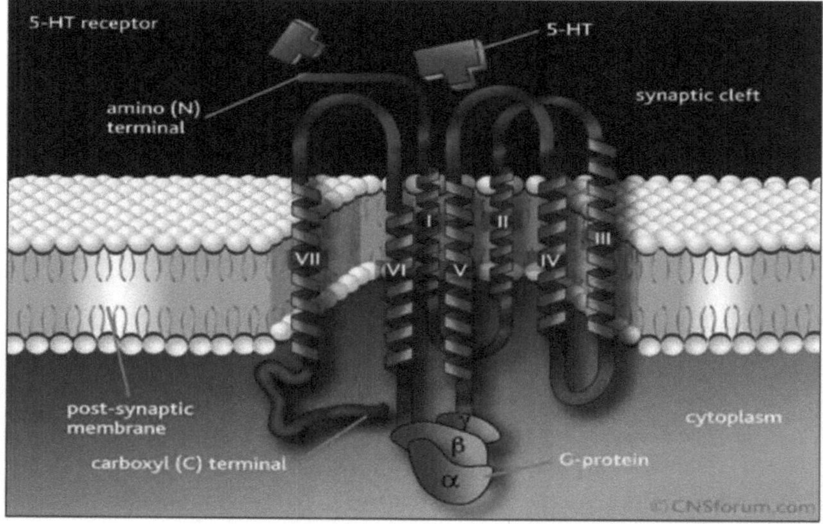

Figure 22: 5-HT1A receptor (http://boundlessthicket.blogspot.com/2012/05/lysergic-acid-diethylamide-and.html)

Play an important role in eating behaviour and the regulation of body temperature. They have been shown to control, at least in part, sexual behaviour and have been implicated in psychiatric disorders such as depression and anxiety (Gerhardt & van Heerikhuizen, 1997). They are widely distributed in the central nervous system in cortico-limbic regions, the hippocampus and the ventral tegmental area (Heisler et al. 1998; Paks, Robinson, Sibille, Shenk, & Toth, 1998).

- **5-Hydroxy-tryptamine2A receptors (coupled to Gaq) :**

The 5-HT2A receptor (471 amino acids) belongs to the superfamily of receptors with 7 G protein-coupled transmembrane domains (GPCRs). Consisting of seven transmembrane domains. The third cytoplasmic loop appears to be involved in coupling with the G protein. When the receptor is activated, the G protein induces a cascade of intracellular reactions involving phospholipase C, which leads to the release of Ca2+ from intracellular storage sites and activation of the MAP kinase pathway.

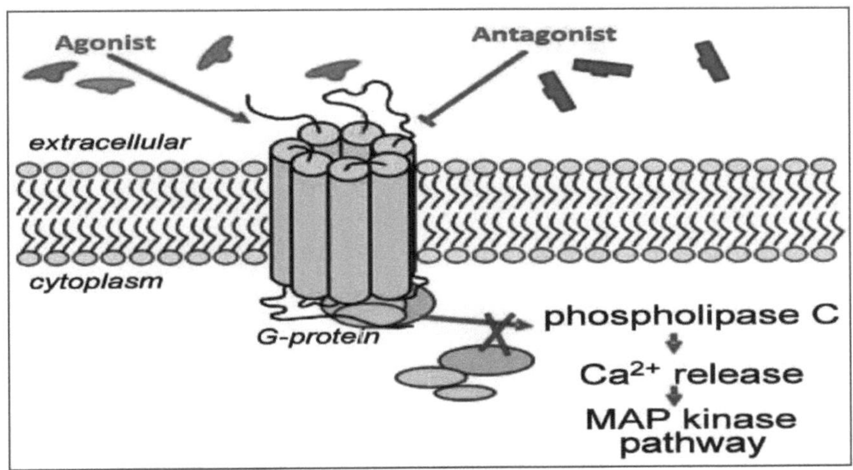

Figure 23: 5-HT2A receptor. (Hoyer et al. 2002)

They are widely distributed in the periphery and in central tissues. Centrally, they are located in limbic structures including the cortex, claustrum, basal ganglia and thalamus. They are involved in psychiatric disorders (such as anxiety, depression, schizophrenia) and in epilepsy, migraine and hallucinations.

In the periphery, they trigger contractile responses in several vascular smooth muscles. They also contribute to platelet aggregation and increased capillary permeability following exposure to serotonin (Hoyer et al. 2002).

b. Signal transduction mechanism :

From the retina to the visual cortical areas, there are synaptic relay zones called the knee bodies. They are made up of different neuronal pathways producing two types of neurotransmitter, serotonin and glutamate.

LSD binds to the 5HT1A receptor on the geniculate body, which induces an increased release of glutamate. The latter binds to excitatory glutamate receptors on the pyramidal neurons of the visual cortex, causing a disruption in the electrical activity of these neurons and a hyper-release.

Next, the release of glutamate activates NMDA receptors which stimulate NADPH oxidase activity, resulting in the production of free radicals, which can be generated by the metabolism of LSD under the action of MPO (myeloperoxidase).

A temporary excess in the production of free radicals can generate UPE (biochemioluminescent photon) in the visual cortex, which induces hallucinations and cognitive disorders. In this case, LSD exerts the same action as serotonin, acting as *a serotonin agonist (G. Kapocs et al/2016).*

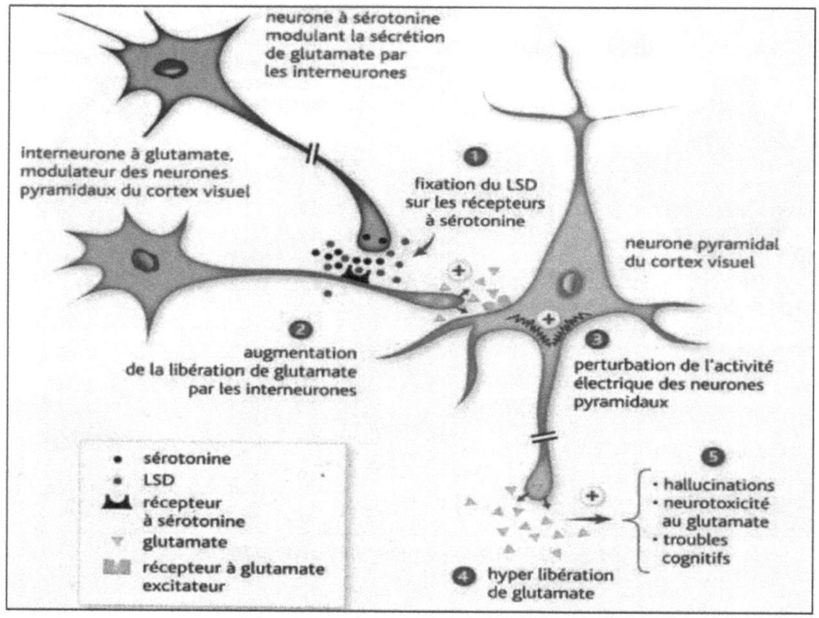

Figure 24: diagram showing the mode of action of LSD (https://clercsvt.jimdo.com/.../1ere-es.../la-chimie-de-la-vision-ses-perturbations)

- **Action of LSD on the reward system :**

The reward system: This is a group of brain structures made up of the nucleus accumbens, the tegmental area, the septum, the hippocampus, the hypothalamus and the prefrontal cortex.

It is essential because it is the seat of the motivation needed to carry out the actions essential to the survival of the species, such as feeding or reproduction. LSD binds to specific serotonin receptors on neurons in the ventral tegmental area, taking the place of serotonin but not activating GABA (inhibitory GABA) neurons like serotonin. As a result, less GABA is released into the synaptic cleft between the GABA neurons and the dopamine neurons, so there is less inhibition, which increases the release of dopamine by the dopaminergic neurons in the nucleus accumbens, the source of the sensation of pleasure. As this release is exacerbated, it leads to euphoria.

It was concluded that LSD plays an antagonistic role to serotonin in the reward circuit. (Olds and Milner, 1954) (www.cache.media.education.fr/).

6. The effect of lysergic acid diethylamides :

a. Short-term effects of LSD :

Consuming LSD can have short-term psychological and physical effects.

- **Psychic effects of LSD :**

LSD causes hallucinations and affects people's brains, causing them to feel things that do not exist but are aware that they are not real, as well as the ability to suddenly recall long-forgotten past events. These memories seem to merge with the present under the effect of LSD. Other effects of LSD may include feelings of weightlessness or heaviness, which may be disconnected from the body, altered ability to judge distance, time or speed, disturbances of speech and vision, and decreased concentration and attention.

Deaths associated with LSD use are usually the result of an accident caused when a person feels or sees something abnormally. This can lead to errors of judgement. For example, users may be convinced that they can fly or cross the street unharmed. (Toronto, 1997)

- **Physical effects of LSD :**

Some of the effects reported by users during and after taking LSD include increased blood pressure and heart rate, increased body temperature or sweating, dizziness, dilated pupils, loss of appetite, nausea or dry mouth, and decreased coordination and weakness.

b. Long-term effects of LSD :

The health risks associated with frequent LSD use are more psychological than physical. The drug can have long-lasting effects on a person's brain and emotional state. Sometimes the effects, such as depression, flashbacks, psychosis and paranoia, continue for years after taking LSD. However, if women take LSD during pregnancy, there may be an increased risk considered to be a toxic effect, such as spontaneous abortions, chromosomal abnormalities in lymphocytes and birth defects in infants.

- **LSD flashbacks**

Some users may experience "flashbacks" after taking LSD. A "flashback" is a recurrence of the effects of the drug without having taken it again. These effects can occur days, weeks or even years after taking LSD.

Although the 'flashbacks' usually diminish over time, they can continue for years. There is currently no established treatment for this disorder and research has not yet conclusively explained the reasons for "flashbacks". (Health Canada, 2000)

- **Psychosis**

Another problem that can develop long after a person has stopped taking LSD is long-term psychosis. Psychosis refers to a loss of contact with reality. Common symptoms include changes in thought patterns (disjointed thinking) delusions of false beliefs that have no basis hallucinations mood changes as well as reduced motivation and loss of interest in life or the future; the user becomes easily discouraged.

CHAPTER 3
CONCLUSION

Cannabis is a plant that has been known since ancient times for its therapeutic properties, but the expansion of its use is mainly for its psychoactive properties, due to the action of cannabinoids, the main components of this plant. It is classified as a substance that disrupts the functioning of the nervous system.

The sensation of mild euphoria, relaxation and heightened auditory and visual perception produced by cannabis is almost entirely explained by its action on cannabinoid receptors. These receptors are present throughout the brain and an endogenous molecule that naturally binds to them, anandamide, has been identified.

Anandamide is involved in regulating mood, memory, appetite, pain, cognition and emotions. When cannabis is introduced into the body, its active ingredient, Delta-9-tetrahydrocannabinol (or THC), can disrupt all these functions.

THC begins by binding to anandamide CB1 receptors. This receptor then modifies the activity of several intracellular enzymes, including cAMP, whose activity it reduces. Less cAMP means less protein kinase A. The reduced activity of this enzyme will affect potassium and calcium channels in such a way as to reduce the quantity of neurotransmitters released. As a result, the general excitability of neuron networks will also be reduced.

However, in the reward circuit, as with other drugs, there is an increase in the release of dopamine. As with opiates, this paradoxical increase is explained by the fact that the dopaminergic neurons in this circuit do not have CB1 receptors but are inhibited by GABAergic neurons, which do. Cannabis therefore lifts the inhibition of GABA neurons and activates dopamine neurons. This increase is at the root of the addiction phenomenon.

Lysergic acid diethylamide is a powerful hallucinogen and is classed as a substance that disrupts the nervous system.

Until 1965, LSD was studied as an adjuvant to psychotherapy and was the subject of numerous publications. A publicity campaign about its toxicity led to it being outlawed and its popularity waning until the late 1990s.

Using LSD can lead to serious and long-lasting psychiatric problems, with users falling into a state of confusion that can be accompanied by anxiety, panic attacks, paranoid disorder, phobias and delirium.

LSD does not cause physical dependence and there is no withdrawal syndrome. It does not stimulate the brain's reward system and has no direct reinforcing effects, i.e. the ability to increase stimulation of pleasure centres located in several brain regions.

Psychological dependence on LSD varies according to the user: a small number of very regular users may experience anxiety or panic when deprived of the drug.

However, the compelling desire to use LSD is in no way comparable to the obsession felt by cocaine or heroin addicts.

References :

- **Abel EL.** Marijuana: The first twelve thousand years. New York: Plénum Press; 1980.

- **Abramson HA**. The use of psychotherapy and alcoholism. Indianapolis, New York, Kansas City: Bobbs Merrill, **1967**

- **Annales** de Toxicologie Analytique, vol. XVI, n° 1, **2004**.

- **Anonymous. Cocaine/Yohimbine** and LSD/Amphetamine mixture in spain. Microgram **2003**; 12: 277.

- **BASTIANIC T., BRISACIER A-C., CADET-TAÏROU A. et al** - Drogues et addictions, données essentielles - OFDT, **2013**, 399p .

- **BECK F., RICHARD J-B** - Les comportements de santé des jeunes - Analyse du Baromètre santé **2010**, INPES, coll. Baromètres santé, 2013, 344 p.

- **Calcagno E, Canetta A, Guzzetti S, Cervo L, Invernizzi RW (2007).** Strain differences in basal and post-citalopram extracellular 5-HT in the mouse medial prefrontal cortex and dorsal hippocampus: relation with tryptophan hydroxylase-2 activity. *J Neurochem* .

- **Campbell VA, Gowran A.** Alzheimer's disease; taking the edge off with cannabinoids? Br J Pharmacol. nov **2007**;152(5):655o 62.

- **Ceglia I, Acconcia S, Fracasso C, Colovic M, Caccia S,Invernizzi RW (2004).** Effects of chronic treatment with escitalopram or citalopram on extracellular 5-HT in the prefrontal cortex of rats: role of 5-HT1A receptors. *Br J Pharmacol* .

- **CHAPARD P.** Hofmann's children. ASUD-Journal, **2008**, n°37, p. 20-21.

- **Clerc D**. Analgesic properties and therapeutic value of cannabis and cannabinoids. Nantes; **2008.**

- **CLERVOY Patrick,** " la petite histoire du LSD ", in Perspective psychiatrique, volume 42, number 2, édition EDK, Paris, p 154-158, **2008**

- **Coscas S.** La revue du praticien : Dossier cannabis. dec **2013**;1419 to 1440.

- **Dahchour A**. Master P2Biomed Neuropharmacology, FSDM. Fez, **2016-2017**

- **De Meijer E. P. M. et al.**(1992), Characterization of Cannabis accessions with regard to cannabinoid content in relation to other plant characteristics,

- **Dr Nuss & Pr Ferreri**, Bichat talks **2001**

- **ELSOHLY M**. Marijuana and the Cannabinoids. Humana Press, Totowa, New Jersey.**2007**. 322p

- **Etiemble J.** Cannabis: what effects on behaviour and health? INSERM; **2001.**

- **Eubanks LM, Rogers CJ, Beuscher AE, Koob GF, Olson AJ, Dickerson TJ, et al.** A molecular link between the active component of marijuana and Alzheimer's disease pathology. Mol Pharm. Dec **2006**;3(6):773 7.

- *Facts About LSD* (fact sheet), Addiction Research Foundation, Toronto, **1997**).

- **G. Kapocs et al**: LSD-induced visual hallucinations and **phosphenes/kapcs2016.**

- **Galland J-P.** Clandestine smoke. Paris (France): Editions du Lézard; **1992**

- **Gerhardt, C. C., & van Heerikhuizen, H.** (1997). Functional characteristics of heterologously expressed 5-HT receptors. *Eur J Pharmacol, 334*(1), 1-23.

- **Goodman, N.** The serotonergic system and mysticism: Could LSD and the nondrug-induced mystical experience share common neural mechanisms? J. Psychoact. Drugs **2002**, 34, 263-272. [CrossRef] [PubMed]

- **Grotenhermen F.** Cannabis in medicine: a practical guide to the medical applications of cannabis and A9-THC. Sélestat: Ed. Indica; **2009.**

- *Hallucinogens* (brochure), Addiction Research Foundation, Toronto, **1997.**

- **Heisler, L. K., Chu, H. M., Brennan, T. J., Danao, J. A., Bajwa, P., Parsons**, L. H., et al. 1998. Elevated anxiety and antidepressant-like responses in serotonin 5- HT1A receptor mutant mice. *Proc Natl Acad Sci U S A, 95*(25), 15049- 15054.

- **Hill R. J.** (1983), Marijuana, Cannabis sativa L., Regulatory Horticulture, Circular No. 5, 9 (12), 57-66.

- **Hoyer, D., Hannon, J. P., & Martin, G. R.** (2002). Molecular, pharmacological and functional diversity of 5-HT receptors. *Pharmacol Biochem Behav, 71*(4), 533-554.

- **Journal de Pharmacie de Belgique** 2002,57, HS 2

- **Julienne M.** Le cannabis: comprendre vite et mieux. Paris: Belin; **2013.**

- **JUNGMANN C.**: LSD: ses utilisations hier et aujourd'hui, Thesis in Pharmacy, Paris V Faculty, **1997.**

- **Drugs** - facts *and* harms, Health Canada, **2000.**

- **Mechoulam, R.**; Hanus, L. A historical overview of chemical research on cannabinoids. Chem. Phys. Lipids, **2000**, 108, 1-13

- Neuroscience **Ed Dale Purves et al**. 3rd Ed. **2004**

- Neurosciences, **2007**, n°5, p. 71-88.

- **Nichols, D. E., & Nichols, C. D.** (2008). Serotonin receptors. Chem Rev, 108(5), 1614-1641.

- **NORTIER E.** Old drugs, new drugs, current practices (Part 2).

- **Ramirez et al**. 2005. Prevention of Alzheimer's disease pathology by cannabinoids. The Journal of Neuroscience 25: 1904-1913.

- **Paris R.R., Moyse H.** Thallophytes in Matière Médicale, Tome I, 2 i , n c Edition. Paris: Masson, **1976**: 328-41.

- **Passie T.** Psycholytic and psychedelic therapy research: A complete international bibliography **1931-1995**. Hannover: Laurentius Publishers, **1997.**

- **Piazza P-V.** Pregnenolone can protect the brain from cannabis intoxication. 2 Jan 2014;343(6166):948.

- **Pierrick. H**, lsd-diethylamide-of-l-lysergic-acid-definition-21696-mxe8ne, **2014**

- Natural protection against cannabis [Internet]. 2014. Available from: http://www.youtube.com/watch?v=GhTJvX18wcs&feature=youtube_gdata_player(accessed September 2014).

- **Richard D, Senon J-L.** Le cannabis: que sais-je? Paris: Presses universitaires de France; **2010.**

- **Savage, C.** Lysergic acid diethylamide (LSD-25) A Clinical-Psychological Study. Am. J. Psychiatry **1952**, 108, 96-900. [CrossRef] [PubMed]

- **Schmid, Y.; Enzler, F.; Gasser, P.; Grouzmann, E.; Preller, K.H.; Vollenweider, F.X.; Brenneisen, R.; Müller, F.; Borgwardt, S.; Liechti, M.E**. Acute effects of lysergic acid diethylamide in healthy subjects. Biol. Psychiatry **2015**, 78, 544-553. [CrossRef] [PubMed]

- **SPILKA S., LE NEZET O., TOVAR M-L.** - Les drogues à 17 ans : premiers résultats de l'enquête ESCAPAD 2011 - OFDT, Février **2012**, Tendance n°79, 4p.

- *Street Drugs:* A Drug Identification Guide, Publishers Group, LLC, Plymouth, MN, **2005**).

- **Tulasne, L.R. (1853)** In: *Annls Sci. Nat.*, Bot. ser. 3 20:45

- **SUGIUDE T., KISHIMOTO S.,OKA S ET AL-Bochimistry** ,pharmacology and physiologie of 2-arachidndlgycerol, an endogenus cannabinoide receptor ligand-progress in lipid research,2006;45:405-446

- **PEREWEE R.G-pharmacology** and therapeutic targets for **A9-tetrahydrocanabinol** and cannabidiol-Euphytica,2004;140:73-81

- **WOOLRIDGE E., BARTON S.-** Cannabis Use in HIV for Pain and other Medical symptoms-jornal of Pain Symptom Management.2005;29

- **Pertwee RG.** Cannabinoid receptors and pain. Prog Neurobiol 2001; 63: 569-611.

Webographic reference :

- www.addictionsuisse.ch/magazine Swiss focus Hallucinogen.

- http://3.bp.blogspot.com/yxoODthzIEU/U1rODITZkwI/AAAAAAAAACU/8zlpLfQZ1kk/s160 0 /cerveau.png

- http://3.bp.blogspot.com/yxoODthzIEU/U1rODITZkwI/AAAAAAAAACU/8zlpLfQZ1kk/s 600/brain.png

- http://tpelsd.e-monsite.com/pages/1 -histoire-du-lsd.html

- http://www.analgesique.wikibis.com/tetrahydrocannabinol.php, (last consulted September **2014**)

- http://www.cannabis-medecin.fr/index.php/formes-consommees (last consulted September **2014**)

- http://www.ipubli.inserm.fr/bitstream/handle/10608/171/? sequence=19

  Accessed on 28 December **2014**

- http://www.nature.com/neuro/journal/v17/n3/full/nn.3647.html

- http://www.vulgaris-medical.com/encyclopedie-medicale/synapse

- https://sensiseeds.com/fr/blog/le-cannabidiol-et-lhuile-de-cbd/

- https://www.alchimiaweb.com/blogfr/cannabis-contre-alzheimer/

- http://carayonbenjamin.wixsite.com/cannabismedecine/action-des-cannaibinoides

- Acces.ens-lyon.fr /acces/resources/neurocienses/reward circuit (olds and milner/1954)

- www.cache.media.education.fr/

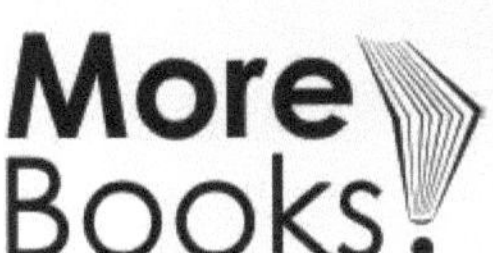

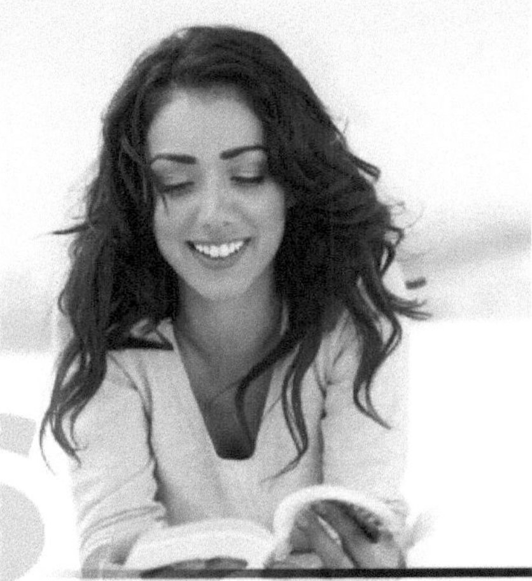

yes
I want morebooks!

Buy your books fast and straightforward online - at one of world's fastest growing online book stores! Environmentally sound due to Print-on-Demand technologies.

Buy your books online at
www.morebooks.shop

Kaufen Sie Ihre Bücher schnell und unkompliziert online – auf einer der am schnellsten wachsenden Buchhandelsplattformen weltweit! Dank Print-On-Demand umwelt- und ressourcenschonend produziert.

Bücher schneller online kaufen
www.morebooks.shop

info@omniscriptum.com
www.omniscriptum.com

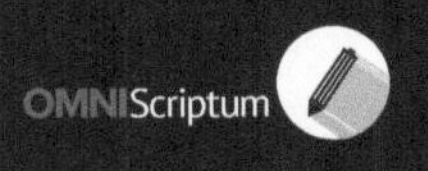

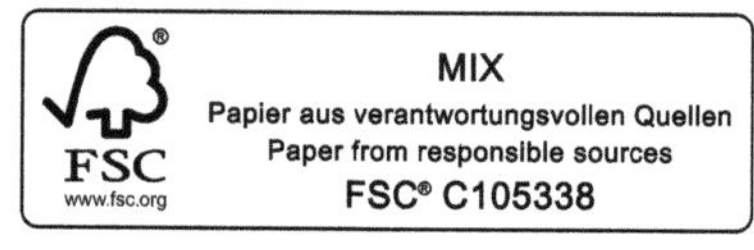

Printed by Books on Demand GmbH, Norderstedt / Germany